THE BLOOD CHOLESTEROL DIET COOKBOOK

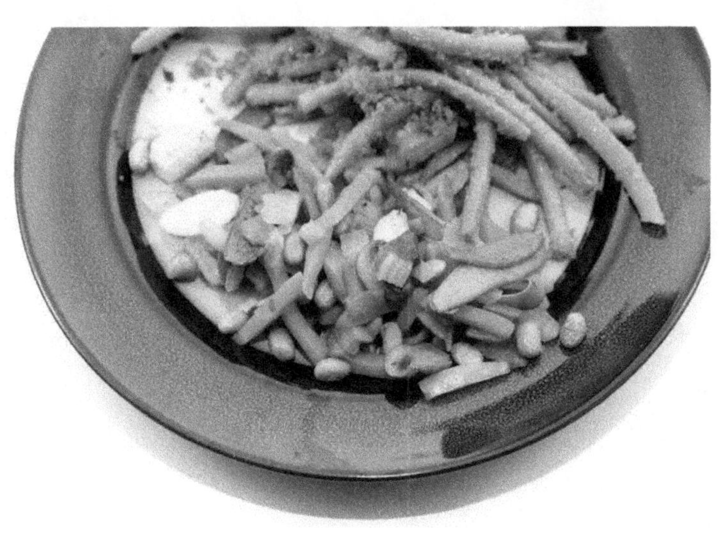

Dr. Penny Watson

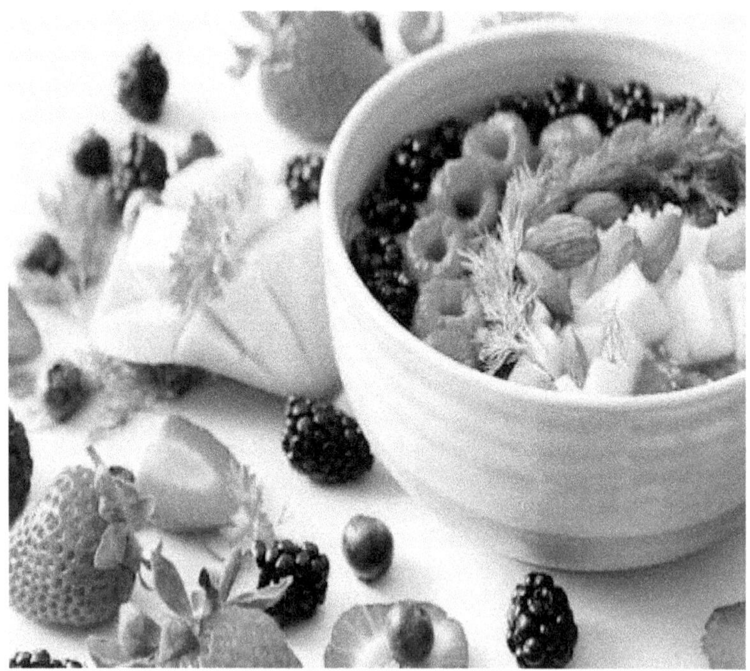

Table of Contents

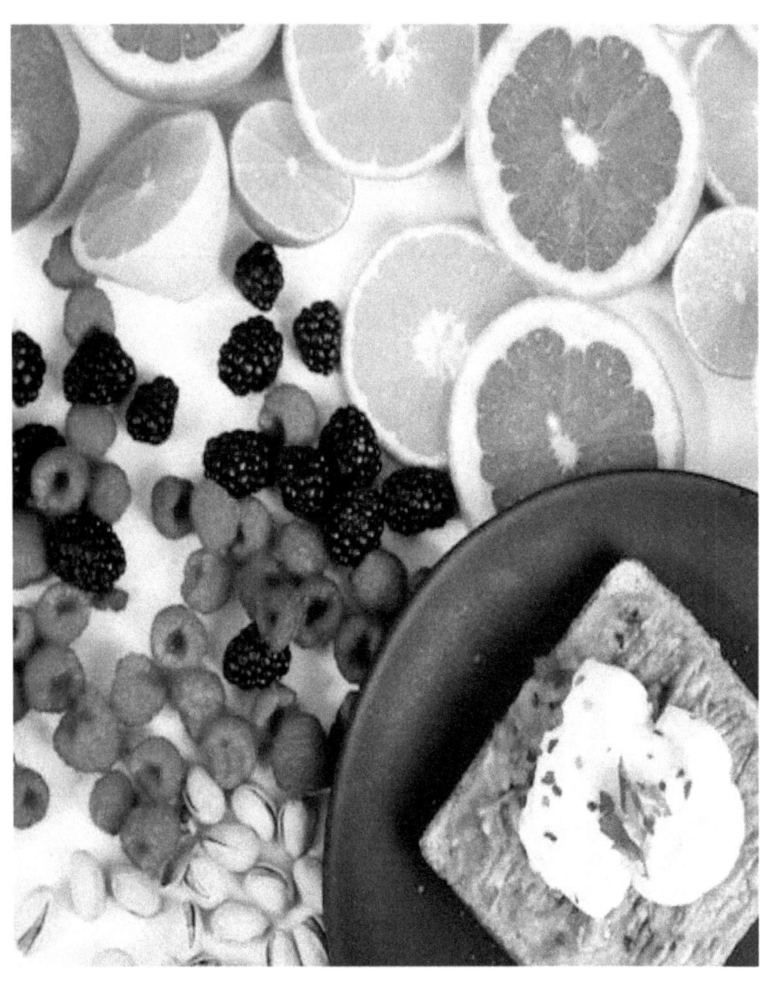

CHAPTER ONE

INTRODUCTION

Managing your high cholesterol (hypercholesteremia) will likely involve a multi-strategy approach, and a diet specifically designed to lower your cholesterol levels is an important one. Advice about what that looks like has changed a bit over the years and, today, it's believed that the foods you choose to eat may matter just as much as (or perhaps more than) those you avoid.

The more high-density lipoprotein (HDL) you have, the more cholesterol your body can remove from your blood. The more low-density lipoprotein (LDL) you have, the more plaque build-up (atherosclerosis) is likely to occur.

The diet recommended to you when you have high cholesterol, then, will involve foods that help increase the former (what's often called "good cholesterol") and decrease the latter (a.k.a., "bad cholesterol"). And perhaps surprisingly, fats and carbohydrates, rather than dietary cholesterol, will be the main focus.

BENEFITS

Your body needs cholesterol for several functions, including forming protective membranes for cells and producing bile to help digest food.

Cholesterol is also used to make vitamin D and hormones like estrogen and testosterone. While diet (meat, eggs, dairy) is a source, cholesterol is also naturally present, as it is made by your liver. Cholesterol plays an important role in your health, but an imbalance of HDL and LDL is of concern. The more HDL you have, the more cholesterol your body can remove from your blood. But if you have a lot of LDL, plaque build-up (atherosclerosis) is more likely to happen, which can lead to heart disease and stroke. Triglycerides, another type of lipid, are fats that you get from your diet that circulate in your blood.

Alcohol, sugar, and excess calories are also converted into triglycerides and stored in body fat. They are also important to note, as they can influence cholesterol levels as well. The diet's biggest benefit can be summed up by the simple fact that it helps give you some ability to manage a condition that has several unmodifiable risk factors, such as family history, age, and sex. The plan takes all of these factors—HDL, LDL, and triglycerides—into account to restore the balance that your body needs to both function and reduce your risk of coronary artery disease (CAD) and other heart diseases.

Fat and carbohydrates in your diet, in combination, are the biggest dietary influences on your cholesterol levels. A diet for high cholesterol focuses on these elements, as well as reducing dietary cholesterol, even though it is not considered as influential as it once was.

Much of the old wisdom on foods to avoid if you have high cholesterol is no longer considered to be accurate, which can lead to some confusion.3 A well-known example is eggs. For many years, eggs were believed to raise cholesterol levels and people with high cholesterol were advised to avoid them.

However, recent research has found that eggs don't have a major influence on cholesterol. In fact, many of the nutritional benefits of eggs can be helpful to people trying to manage their cholesterol with diet.

While each person's body is uniquely sensitive to the cholesterol, they get from the food they eat, research indicates that the influence of dietary cholesterol on cholesterol levels is noteworthy, but mild compared to other factors. The fact that all fats are not equal plays a role here, too. While saturated fats can negatively affect lipid levels (specifically, LDL), healthy fats, such as those found in nuts and avocado, can help lower cholesterol levels by boosting your HDL.

Everyone Is Different

Although you can make decisions about your diet, you can't control how your body responds to cholesterol in the food you eat. Research has indicated that some people are naturally more sensitive to it than others, and the cholesterol levels of "responders" are more influenced by diet than those of "non-responders." For people who aren't as sensitive, what they eat doesn't influence their levels much (if at all). There are several treatments for high cholesterol and you may need to simultaneously use more than one to get your levels down and keep them in a healthy range.

How it works

When you're thinking about how much cholesterol is in your diet, remember that your body makes its own supply—and it will provide what you need, despite your diet. As such, there isn't a set amount of cholesterol you need to get from the food you eat. In the past, the general recommendation was 300 milligrams (mg) of dietary cholesterol (or less) per day. However, in 2018, the American Heart Association guidelines for dietary cholesterol intake were changed. Most adults, whether they have high cholesterol or not, are advised to keep dietary cholesterol intake low while still eating a varied, balanced, and "heart-healthy" diet, but adherence to these guidelines is especially important if you've been prescribed a diet for high cholesterol. Your healthcare provider may make more specific recommendations for you based on your overall health (for example, if you have other chronic health conditions or risk factors for heart disease).

Duration

Once you've made changes to the way you eat to help manage your cholesterol, you'll likely need to keep those changes long term; going back to your previous diet may encourage your levels to rise again. Given this, it may help to think about your new way of eating as a permanent lifestyle modification rather than a temporary diet.

Recommended timing

In 2019, researchers reviewed the findings from the Nutrition and Health Survey in Taiwan to see if the timing of meals had any specific impact on cholesterol levels. The research indicated people who ate more at night may have higher LDL cholesterol levels than people who ate most of their food during the day. When these individuals consumed what would normally be their late-day calories earlier in the day instead, they had lower cholesterol levels.

Another group of researchers looked at whether skipping meals had an effect on cholesterol levels.

The research found people who skipped breakfast had higher LDL cholesterol, and people who skipped dinner had more triglycerides and a higher ratio of total and HDL cholesterol.

CHAPTER TWO

Cooking Tips

As you're preparing meals, you can reduce the fat content of meat by:

• Selecting lean cuts of meat with no visible fat

• Trimming remaining fat or gristle from meat and removing the skin before serving

• Grilling, broiling, or roasting meat rather than frying it with high-fat butter or oil

With fruits and vegetables, avoid adding salt, sugar, butter, or canola oil, which are high in trans fats. To avoid diminishing their nutritional power, avoid adding any sweet sauces, fat, or grease to beans and legumes.

Instead, add flavour with spices. Aside from being tasty, many popular herbs and spices have properties that can change how LDL cholesterol interacts with free radicals—particles that can make the molecules in LDL unstable, causing inflammation and further impacting your cardiovascular health.

The antioxidants in some fresh herbs and spices have been shown to prevent these damaging interactions.

Garlic is another healthy and versatile option for savory meals that can help lower cholesterol and triglyceride levels.

When baking, try adding ginger, allspice, and cinnamon, all of which are high in antioxidants. Instead of making baked goods using lard, butter, or oil, try using substitutes like applesauce, banana, or even avocado.

Modifications

Again, the diet recommended for you will be tailored to your condition and overall health profile. Your healthcare provider may suggest a stricter plan for you, for example, if you have several compounding risk factors at play.

Even still, sometimes changing how you eat may not be enough to lower your cholesterol.

Adding other lifestyle modifications like increasing your physical activity and losing weight may also prove insufficient.

If your levels are still high on a low cholesterol diet, your practitioner may prescribe statins, medications that would be taken as you continue on with your diet for high cholesterol.

Considerations

If you're planning to make changes to your diet, it's important to consider all the different parts of your life that might be affected. Your lifestyle, responsibilities, and preferences also influence your ability to make (and stick to) the changes you make.

General Nutrition

Compared to diets that heavily restrict which foods you can eat, a diet for high cholesterol can be quite varied and balanced.

Fresh produce, lean meats, and low-fat dairy are all approved on this plan and part of a healthy diet for anyone.

Many of the foods you may want to avoid or limit on a low-cholesterol diet are high in fat, sugar, and calories. Choosing not to include these foods in your diet (or having them only in moderation) can have health benefits beyond managing cholesterol, such as helping you lose weight or lower your blood pressure.

FLEXIBILITY

Though you may need to expand your typical shopping list and modify some favourite recipes, the wide range of foods that are appropriate on a diet for high cholesterol make the plan quite flexible. Many restaurant menus highlight heart-healthy or low-fat selections, which may be appropriate.

You can also ask to make simple swaps like a whole-grain wrap instead of a bun, or grilled chicken instead of fried.

DIETARY RESTRICTIONS

If you're not sure how to make your dietary needs and preferences work with a low-cholesterol diet, you may want to talk with a registered dietitian or nutritionist. They can guide you through creating a lipid-lowering meal plan.

Such advice can be particularly helpful if you are also managing a gastrointestinal concern that is worsened by fiber/roughage or you need to avoid gluten (millet, teff, and quinoa are choices that are safe and packed with fiber).

Side Effects

By itself, a cholesterol-lowering diet shouldn't have any side effects. Whenever you make changes to how you eat, it's possible you will experience temporary bowel symptoms such as constipation, but these are usually temporary and get better as you adjust. If you are starting a cholesterol-lowering drug as well, remember that any side effects you experience could also be the result of your medication. For example, muscle pain and weakness are common side effects of statins. Speak to your healthcare provider about anything you're experiencing that is of concern.

General Health

The foods recommended to manage high cholesterol offer a myriad of other health benefits. Two in particular—helping you maintain a healthy weight and improving your energy—can make other changes, like exercising more, easier to adopt. This can obviously help your cholesterol-lowering efforts, but it will also help reduce your risk of issues beyond cardiovascular ones, including cancer.

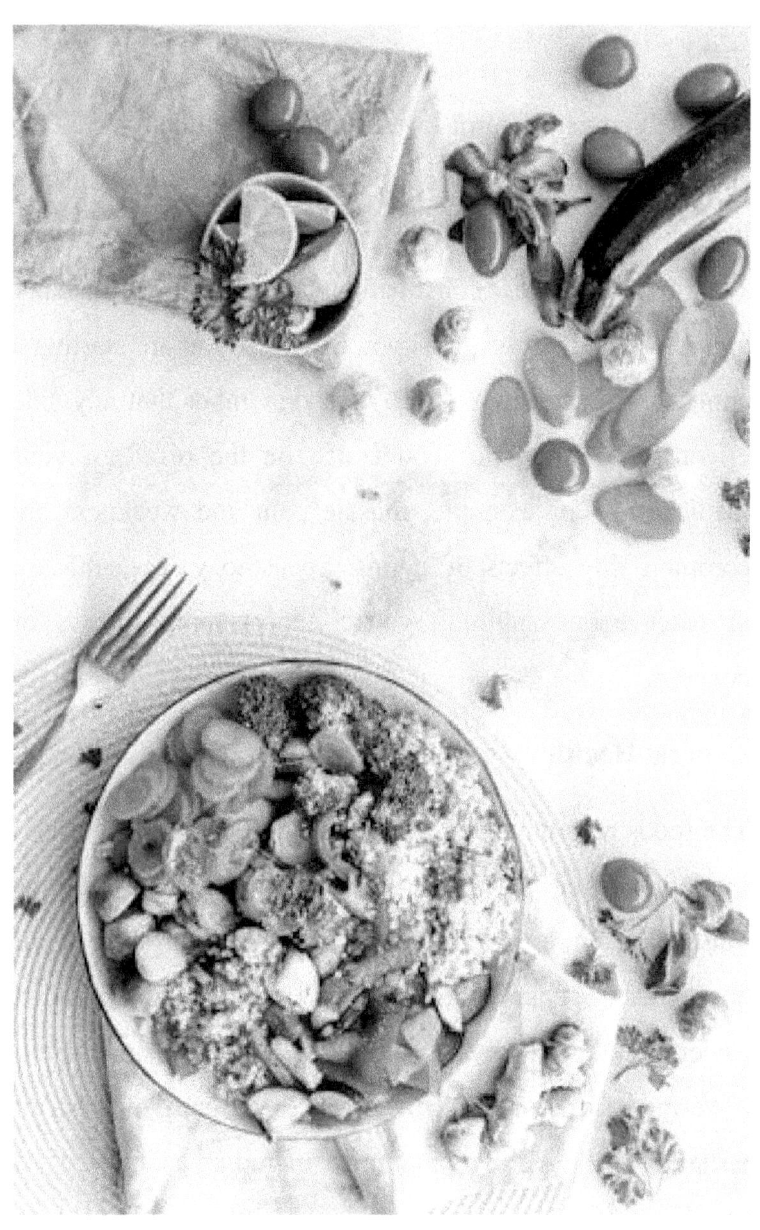

CHAPTER THREE

TIPS FOR FOLLOWING A LOW CHOLESTEROL DIET

Prepare Your Kitchen

The first step you can take towards incorporating a lipid-lowering diet into your healthy lifestyle is to stock your kitchen with heart-healthy foods.

Start by throwing out or donating foods that are high in saturated fat and refined sugars. These foods are high in calories and can adversely affect your lipid levels.

Foods to exclude from your kitchen include:

• High-sugar soft drinks

• Potato chips

• Cookies

• Candy

• Fried foods

• Pastries

Remember, if these foods aren't available, you can't eat them! Consider limiting these foods to special occasions only, if you eat them at all.

If you must keep these foods in the house for other family members, place them behind healthy foods in your cabinet or refrigerator. That way, if you become tempted to reach for unhealthy foods, you will see healthy foods first.

Despite some of the foods you are eliminating from your diet, there are plenty of cholesterol-friendly foods you can include, such as:

• Vegetables

• Fruit

• Fish

• Legumes

• Nuts

• Seeds

• Whole grain products

Get to Know Your Grocery Store

With the wide selection of foods, grocery shopping can sometimes get quite overwhelming when starting a lipid-lowering diet and this can place you at risk of resorting back to your tried-and-true, unhealthy foods.

To get around this, you should always create a list of healthy foods you would like to eat before going to the grocery store and stick to it.

If you do not like to make lists, you can select cholesterol-friendly foods by "shopping the perimeter." Fresh fruits and vegetables, lean meats, and low-fat dairy products are found in the outside aisles of the grocery store, while packaged and processed foods are stored in the interior aisles.

Purchase two fresh fruits or vegetables that you have not tried before or have not had in a while. Fresh fruits and vegetables, such as apples, berries, bananas, carrots, and broccoli, are an important source of soluble fiber, which can lower your LDL cholesterol levels.

For packaged foods, start looking at snacks and meals with health claims of "high-fiber" or "whole-grain" and begin to look at the nutrition facts label listed on the product. Don't feel that you have to completely understand the information listed on the nutrition label right away; just get in the habit of looking at it for now.

Research Restaurants

Eating out is sometimes another source of added fat and calories to your lipid-lowering diet. To make your dining experience a more cholesterol-friendly one, you may need to do a little research before you go out to eat. Go online and look at the menus of restaurants you visit often, as well as new restaurants that you have not tried before.

Look for heart-healthy or vegetarian icons next to foods, and consider trying some of these dishes the next time you dine out.

Some restaurants will also list calorie, saturated fat, and carbohydrate content of the food - which is also helpful when planning your meals.

Getting in the habit of checking out a restaurant's menu before you dine will help you to cut calories from your meal when you eat out and avoid potentially unhealthy foods.

Try Healthier Cooking Techniques

If you opt to make your own meals instead of eating out, there are some ways you can make your foods more heart-healthy. By using the following cooking techniques, you can cut out fat and calories from your dish:

• Baking

• Broiling

• Roasting

• Steaming

• Grilling

• Boiling

You should avoid frying your foods since this can introduce extra saturated fat and unhealthy trans fats to your meal.

Healthy Snacking on a Low Cholesterol Diet

A good low cholesterol diet contains a lot of cholesterol-lowering foods - whether you have the time to cook a full course meal or have just enough time to grab and go.

Having too many things to do and too .little time on your hands, eating healthy may be low on the list of your priorities.

On some days, full course meals are neglected in favour of quicker, lighter snacks. Let's face it--snacking is natural. If you are hungry between meals, your body is telling you that it needs nutrition now.

Therefore, you should definitely eat something to curb your hunger until the next meal.

Eating the wrong snacks, however, is what can get you into trouble.

Snacks high in fats and carbohydrates can increase cholesterol levels, cause weight gain, and can eventually lead to complications such as heart disease, high cholesterol, and diabetes.

The good news is that, with so many people concerned with eating healthy these days, many food manufacturers have developed low fat, low carbohydrate alternatives to foods that are almost identical in taste to the "real thing".

When grazing for food, keep these things in mind

Eat Plenty of Fruits and Vegetables They are low in calories and fat.

Additionally, they contain a number of vitamins and other antioxidants that prevent cellular damage and aid in a number of cellular processes.

Watch Your Saturated Fat Intake

Consumption of saturated fats should be limited, if not avoided, since they are associated with raising cholesterol levels.

Saturated fats are usually encountered in fried foods and in animal meats.

On a side note, concerning animal meats: lean meats, such as chicken, fish, and turkey are less in saturated fat than red meat.

Watch What You Put on the Food That You Cook

Partially hydrogenated vegetable oils, such as those used in many margarines and shortenings, contain a particular form of fat known as trans-fatty acids.

These should also be avoided since they raise cholesterol levels.

They are usually found in fried foods and processed foods, such as cookies, chips, and candies.

Dips and Toppings Restrictions

If you need to use salad dressing, sauces, or dips, try a low-fat alternative. Also, use them on the side instead of placing them directly on your food--you will use a lot less this way.

Try Low-Fat Varieties of Your Favourite Dairy Products

Selecting low-fat dairy products will also help to lower fat consumption instead of their "full strength" counterparts.

An example of this would be to substitute low-fat yogurt or non-fat milk instead of regular milk or yogurt.

Carbohydrates Are an Important and Quick Energy Source

Since these are converted to sugar in the body, consumption of too many carbohydrates can cause weight gain and elevated glucose levels in diabetics.

Additionally, previous research has indicated that consuming too many carbohydrates can lower HDL (good cholesterol) levels.

Whole grain products, such as wheat bread and oats, are low in flour and high in fiber, minerals, and vitamins.

With the gaining popularity of the Atkins diet, many food manufacturers have low-carbohydrate versions of bread and other grains. Low fat, unsalted pretzels, and unbuttered, unsalted popcorn are also good alternatives.

Nuts and Seeds (Preferably Unsalted) Are Good and Filling Snack Foods

They contain large amounts of unsaturated fats, and unsaturated fats tend to lower total cholesterol levels.

Nuts (especially walnuts) contain omega 3-fatty acids, which have been linked to lowering total and LDL (low-density lipoprotein—the "bad" cholesterol) cholesterol levels while raising HDL (high-density lipoprotein—the "good" cholesterol) cholesterol levels.

Seeds, including pumpkin and sunflower seeds, contain high amounts of Vitamin E, B vitamins, and minerals.

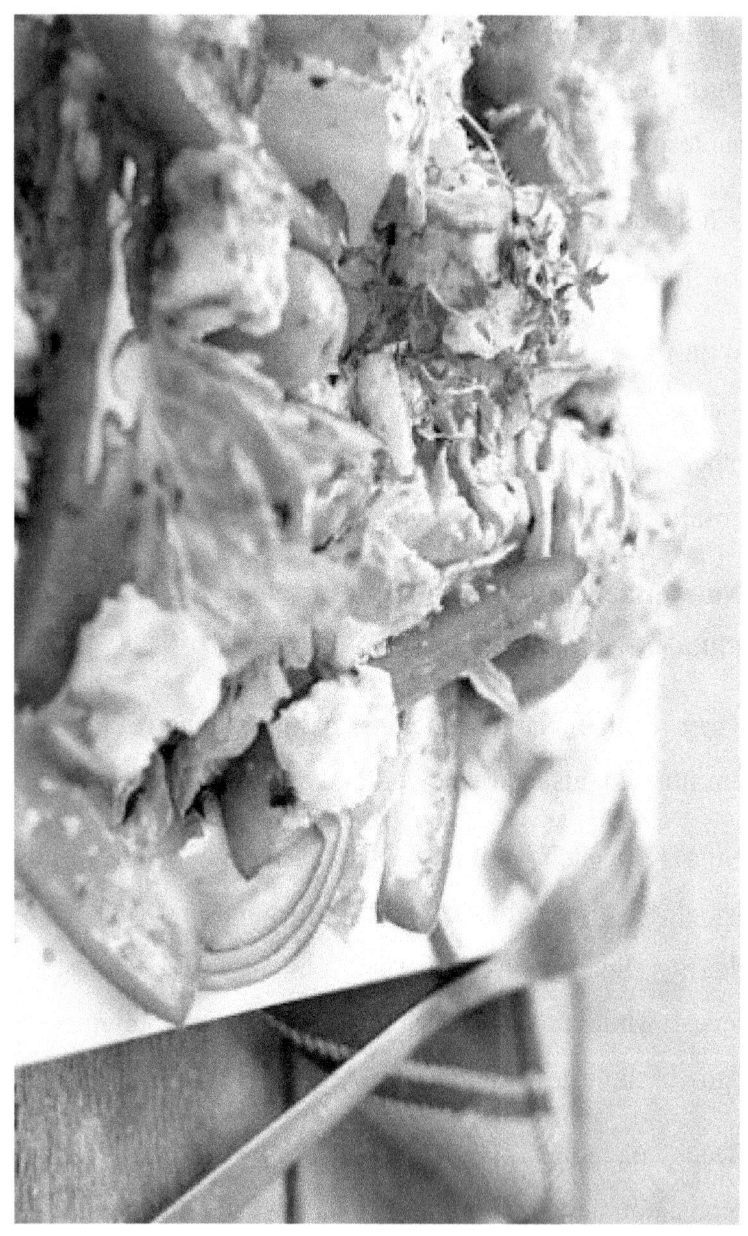

CHAPTER FOUR

LOW CHOLESTEROL RECIPES

1. Low Cholesterol Chicken Meatloaf

INGREDIENTS

• 1 lb ground chicken, or any lean ground meat like chuck or turkey

• 2 cups oats, quick-cooking

• 11 oz marinara sauce, divided

• 3 oz red onion, minced

• 2 oz bell peppers, of your choice, minced

• 1½ oz carrots, minced

• salt, to taste

• ground black pepper, to taste

To Serve:

• 1½ cups potato, fried

• 4 oz vegetables, (green beans, onions, and tomatoes), pan-grilled

• parsley

INSTRUCTIONS

1. Preheat the oven to 350 degrees F. Grease a loaf tin and baking sheet with cooking spray.

2. In a bowl, combine the ground chicken, 7 ounces of marinara sauce, onions, bell peppers, carrots, and oats in a bowl.

3. Season with salt and pepper, then mix all the ingredients together, then transfer into the greased loaf pan.

4. Cover with foil, then transfer to the oven. Bake for 1 hour, or until meatloaf is fully cooked.

5. Once baked, remove and discard the foil.

Pour off any excess liquid or fat, then invert onto your greased baking sheet.

6. Pour over the remaining marinara sauce and spread to cover the meatloaf.

Return back to the oven and broil until the sauce glazes the meatloaf.

7. Portion accordingly, serve with potatoes and vegetables done your way, then garnish with parsley. Enjoy!

RECIPE NOTES

• If you feel like the mixture is not thick enough, you can add more oats until you achieve your desired consistency.

2. Chilled Avocado Soup

INGREDIENTS

• 3 avocados, ripe, pitted and peeled; or 1½ lb frozen avocado pulp, thawed

• 7 oz cucumber, deseeded and chopped, unpeeled.

• 1 lime, juiced

• 3 cups plant-based milk, of your choice, preferably almond milk, except coconut, used soy milk.

• ½ cup cilantro, with stems and leaves, chopped

• 1 cup peanuts, roasted

• salt and ground black pepper, to taste

To Serve:

• cilantro leaves

INSTRUCTIONS

1. Combine the avocado, cucumber, milk, cilantro, and peanuts in a food processor or blender except for the lime juice, salt, and pepper.

2. Puree until smooth, then adjust the seasoning with salt and pepper.

Add the lime juice and blend briefly.

3. Portion into preferred glassware's. Garnish with cilantro, serve, and enjoy!

3. Broccoli Almond

INGREDIENTS

• 2 lb broccoli, florets only

• ½ cup butter, unsalted

• ½ cup almonds, flaked, sliced, slivered or roasted

• 2 cloves garlic, minced

• 1½ tbsp corn-starch

• 1½ cup chicken broth

• salt, to taste

• pepper, to taste

INSTRUCTIONS

1. Heat up a wide skillet over medium heat and melt butter.

2. Add garlic & sauté until golden.

3. Add broccoli and sauté until tender.

4. Dissolve corn-starch in chicken broth.

Mix to combine then add broth to broccoli.

Boil just until thickened.

5. Add the almonds then toss to combine.

6. Season with salt and pepper to taste. Adjust accordingly.

7. Serve with mashed potatoes roughly 1 cup per serving.
Best with chicken.

4. Bean Salad With Pine Nuts and Feta

INGREDIENTS

• 15 oz red kidney beans, (1 can), drained and rinsed

• 15 oz pinto beans, (1 can), drained and rinsed

• 7 oz cucumber, peeled, seeded, and chopped

• 4 oz bell peppers, preferably a mix of colours and chopped

• 1½ oz red onion, finely chopped

• ¼ cup parsley, finely chopped

• 3 tbsp balsamic vinegar

• 2 tbsp olives, pitted and sliced, preferably cured

• 2 tbsp feta cheese, crumbled

• 2 tbsp pine nuts, roasted

• 1½ tbsp olive oil

• 1 tbsp apple cider vinegar

• 1 tsp Dijon mustard

• 1 tsp honey

• salt and ground black pepper, to taste

INSTRUCTIONS

1. In a small bowl, make the dressing by whisking together both kinds of vinegar, olive oil, mustard, and honey.

2. Season with salt and pepper. Adjust accordingly. Whisk until emulsified and set aside.

3. In a large salad bowl, combine both beans, cucumbers, bell peppers, onions, parsley, olives, feta cheese, and pine nuts.

4. Drizzle dressing on the salad and toss well. Adjust seasoning as needed and serve.

5. Sugar-Free Apple Pie

INGREDIENTS

• 2 tsp tapioca, or corn-starch flour

• 1 tsp ground cinnamon, or nutmeg

• ½ cup apple cider

• 4 cups green apples, sliced

• 20 oz pie crust dough, prepared, divided into 2 large discs

• 1 egg yolk

• 1 tbsp milk

• all-purpose flour, for dusting

INSTRUCTIONS

1. Preheat your oven to 325 degrees F.

2. Assemble the filling by combining tapioca flour, cinnamon, apple cider, and apples together. Mix until evenly incorporated and set aside.

3. Dust both your rolling pin and working area with flour.

4. Roll out 1 disc of dough until you achieve a roughly ½ inch thickness.

5. Transfer the dough onto your greased pie tin. Leave excess dough hanging on the sides of the pie tin.

6. Pour your filling onto your pie tin.

7. Repeat steps with remaining dough.

8. Cover the pie and seal edges.

Then, make a few slits on top.

9. Prepare your egg wash by beating together egg yolk and milk.

10. Brush this around and on top of your pie.

11. Bake for roughly 40 minutes, then increase your oven temperature to 400°F.

Broil the crush until golden, roughly 10 minutes.

12. Allow to cool down and serve.

6. Citrus Glazed Salmon with Pecan-Citrus Rice

INGREDIENTS

For Orange Salmon Glaze:

- ¾ cup honey

- ¾ cup orange juice

- 1 tsp whole black peppercorns, cracked

- 1 whole star anise pod

- 2 tbsp orange zest

• 2 tbsp lemon zest

• 2 tbsp grapefruit zest

For Pecan-Citrus Rice:

• 1 cup long grain rice

• ¾ cup orange juice

• ¾ cup water

• ¼ cup parsley, chopped

• ½ cup pecans, chopped and toasted

• salt and ground black pepper, to season

For Salmon Fillets:

• 4 salmon fillets, (about 4 oz each), skinless

• salt and ground black pepper, to season

• 2 tbsp vegetable oil

To Serve:

• parsley sprigs

INSTRUCTIONS

Orange Salmon Glaze:

1. Preheat the oven to 400 degrees F. Grease a baking sheet with cooking spray, line with parchment paper, and grease again with cooking spray.

2. Combine the peppercorns, star anise, honey, orange juices, lemon zest, and orange zest in a saucepot. Bring to a boil, then reduce to a simmer.

Continue simmering for at least 20 minutes, or until it is reduced by half and slightly thickened.

3. Once the glaze has thickened, remove from the heat and set aside to steep for another 15 minutes, then strain and discard all solids. Set aside to cool down completely.

Pecan-Citrus Rice:

1. Cook your rice next. Combine the rice, water, and orange juice in your rice cooker. Boil until your rice is cooked through, following the manufacturer's instructions. This will be anywhere from 20 to 30 minutes.

Salmon Fillets:

1. While the rice is cooking, heat up a skillet with oil over medium-high heat. Add the salmon, season with salt and pepper. Sear on all sides until golden brown, roughly 3 minutes per side.

2. Layer your seared salmon fillets inches apart from each other onto a lined baking sheet.

3. Brush your glaze all over the salmon fillets, then roast in the oven for roughly 5 to 8 minutes, until the salmon just starts flaking and the glaze has turned golden.

4. Baste with the glaze as needed while roasting.

5. Once roasted, set aside onto cooling racks and allow to rest briefly.

6. Once your rice is cooked, transfer it into a mixing bowl. Add pecans and parsley and mix until combined.

7. Season with salt and ground pepper to taste and adjust accordingly. Mix to combine.

8. Serve your salmon with 1 cup of pecan-citrus rice.

Garnish with parsley roughly ¼ teaspoon parsley and enjoy.

7. Barley-Herb Casserole

INGREDIENTS

• 3¾ oz pearl barley

• 3 tbsp fresh parsley, preferably flat leaf, minced

• ¼ tsp dried rosemary

• 4 oz chickpeas, canned, drained

• 2 cups vegetable broth

• 1 tsp vegetable oil

• 1 cup squash, or pumpkin, diced

• 5½ oz red onion, chopped

• 1 medium tomato

• salt, to taste

• freshly ground black pepper, to taste

To Serve:

• 1 tbsp parmesan cheese, grated or powdered, per serving

• ¼ tbsp parsley, chopped, per serving

INSTRUCTIONS

1. Preheat the oven to 350 degrees F.

2. Heat up the oil in a skillet over medium heat. Add the onion, squash, and rosemary. Sauté for 6 to 7 minutes, stirring frequently, until the vegetables are slightly caramelized.

3. Add the barley and continue sauteing until the mixture is thoroughly combined.

4. Remove from heat, then stir in the tomato, chickpeas, and parsley.

5. Season with salt and pepper, stir to combine, then transfer the barley mixture to a baking dish. Add the broth.

6. Cover with foil, then bake for 1 hour.

7. Remove the foil and continue baking for 15 more minutes until the liquid is absorbed and the mixture is heated through.

8. Portion accordingly, garnish with parmesan cheese and parsley. Have your guests help themselves with either marinara sauce or pesto for another depth of flavour. Serve and enjoy!

8. Oatmeal with Fresh Blueberries

INGREDIENTS

- 1⅓ cup water

- ¼ tsp ground cinnamon

- 1 tbsp honey

- ⅔ cup oatmeal

- ⅓ cup blueberries, fresh

- ½ tsp orange zest, finely minced

- ½ cup coconut milk, or plant-based milk of your choice, preferably almond milk

INSTRUCTIONS

1. Boil water in a medium-size saucepan, then stir in the cinnamon, honey, and oatmeal. Reduce the heat to simmering and cook for five minutes.

2. Stir in the orange zest and milk.

3. Stir occasionally and simmer for five more minutes or until the oatmeal is thick and creamy.

4. Cool down for five minutes, then serve topped with fresh blueberries.

9. Chocolate Orange Fondue

INGREDIENTS

• 12 oz dark chocolate, or white chocolate, bars or chips, shaved if using bars

• 1¼ cups heavy cream

• 1 cup orange liqueur

• orange juice, from 1 orange

• orange zest, from 1 orange

• salt, to taste

To Serve:

• your choice of accompaniments

INSTRUCTIONS

1. Combine orange liqueur and orange juice in a saucepot. Bring to a boil over medium heat.

2. Continue boiling until most of the alcohol has evaporated and is almost syrupy, roughly 10 minutes. Set aside at room temperature to cool completely.

3. Heat the cream in a saucepan over medium heat until it starts to bubble at the edges.

4. Remove from the heat, and immediately whisk in the chocolate, orange zest, and cooled down orange syrup until smooth.

5. Adjust seasoning with salt to balance out the sweetness.

6. Serve immediately with your choice of accompaniments, preferably in a fondue pot over the lowest heat setting, or farthest from the heat source.

10. Armenian Stuffed Eggplant

INGREDIENTS

• 2 eggplants, roughly 2 lb total, medium, sliced in half

- 8 oz yellow onions, small dice

- 2 cloves garlic, minced

- ¼ tsp red chili flakes

- ¼ tsp ground cinnamon

- 12 oz tomatoes, de-seeded and cut into small dice

- 1 tsp granulated sugar

- 2 tbsp parsley, fresh, finely chopped, and divided

- 2 tbsp lemon juice, fresh

- ¼ tsp salt, plus extra for the eggplant

- ½ cup olive oil

To serve:

- 1 tbsp parsley, chopped

INSTRUCTIONS

1. Using a knife, make slits down the middle of the eggplants. Make sure not to slice too deeply till you slice through them.

2. Lightly salt the eggplant slices and leave it for 20 minutes. Pat them dry then set them aside.

3. Heat olive oil in a large saucepan over medium-high heat and add the eggplants, cut side down. Add more oil as needed.

4. Fry gently until cut sides turn golden brown. Flip over and fry the skin until it starts to shrivel.

Remove eggplants from the pan and let them drain on paper towels for 15 minutes.

Save the remaining olive oil for later.

5. Preheat the oven to 350 degrees F.

6. Sauté the onions over medium heat for 5 minutes then add in the garlic, red chili flakes, salt, and cinnamon.

Cook for 1-minute then pour in the tomatoes and let it simmer for 5 minutes to let it thicken. Remove from the heat and stir in 1 tablespoon of parsley.

7. Spoon the onion and tomato mixture in between the slits of each eggplant.

8. Brush the stuffed eggplants with lemon juice. Sprinkle your eggplants with sugar.

9. Cover it with foil and bake your dish in the oven for roughly 45 minutes, or until the eggplant is already tender and the sauce has caramelized.

10. Once your dish is done baking, let it sit for 10 minutes before cutting your eggplant slices.

11. Garnish it with parsley and enjoy your flavourful meat-free dish. You also have the option to serve this whole as a main course.

11. Lentil And Chestnut Soup

INGREDIENTS

- ½ lb dry lentils

- 16 chestnuts, coarsely crumbled, cooked

- 2 tbsp. olive oil

- 1 onion, diced

- ¼ tsp cinnamon

- 1 bay leaf

• 1 tsp fresh thyme, chopped

• 4 cups water, vegetable, meat or poultry stock

• 2 tbsp tomato paste

• salt

• fresh black pepper

• fried bread croutons, optional for garnish

• 3 tbsp parsley, chopped

• 1 tbsp fresh thyme, chopped

INSTRUCTIONS

1. Soak the lentils in water to cover for a few hours or overnight (12 hours).

2. Melt the pancetta fat and cook the onion over moderate heat until tender, about 8 minutes, adding salt and a little cinnamon if desired. (The cinnamon will play up the sweetness of the onion, pancetta and chestnuts.)

3. Add the lentils, bay leaf, thyme and water or stock, and bring up to a boil.

4. Reduce the heat and simmer until the lentils are tender but not falling apart.

5. Add the tomato paste and chestnuts and simmer for 5 minutes.

6. Season to taste with salt and pepper.

7. Garnish with fried bread croutons if desired, and chopped parsley and thyme.

12. Low-Fat Trifle

INGREDIENTS

• 1 ½ cup cold fat free milk

• 1 ½ oz JELL-O Vanilla Flavour Fat Free Sugar Free Instant Reduced Calorie Pudding & Pie Filling, (4-serving size)

• 8 oz Cool Whip Lite Whipped Topping, thawed & divided

• 13 oz angel food cake, cut into 1/2-inch cubes (about 6-1/2 cups)

• 2 cups strawberries, sliced

• 1 cup blueberries

INSTRUCTIONS

1. Beat pudding mix and milk in medium bowl with whisk 2 min.

2. Stir in 1-1/2 cups COOL WHIP.

3. Layer half each of the cake and berries in large serving bowl; cover with pudding mixture.

4. Top with layers of remaining cake, berries and COOL WHIP.

5. Refrigerate 1 hour.

6. You're ready to serve!

13. Chicken Fajitas

INGREDIENTS

• 16ozchicken strip cooked

• orange bell pepper julienned

• ½ red bell pepper julienned

• ½ green bell pepper julienned

- ½ white onion julienned

- 1cuplow sodium chicken broth

- 2cupsquinoacooked

- 1tbspmongolian sauce

- 1tspolive oil

- ½ onion julienned

For Seasoning:

- 1lemonjuiced

- 1tsppepper

- ½ scalene pepper

- ½ tspred chili flakes

- ½ tspsalt

- ½ tspgarlic powder

- ½ tsponion powder

INSTRUCTIONS

1. Mix chicken strips with seasonings and lemon juice and set aside.

2. Heat olive oil in a medium pan on medium heat and add the garlic, sautéing for about 1 minute. Quickly add the chicken broth and stir to avoid burning the garlic.

3. Add in the chicken and peppers, cover and cook on medium for about 5 minutes.

4. Then, add onion and remove from heat once the broth is bubbling and the peppers look fully cooked.

5. Mix Mongolian sauce with quinoa.

6. Serve chicken and veggies alongside prepared quinoa.

14. Mill Cottage's Ultimate High Fiber Oatmeal

INGREDIENTS

• 1 1/2 cup water

• 1/4 tsp salt

• 1/3 cup oatmeal, or equal parts of steel cut oats, old fashioned

• 1/3 cup barley

• rye

• wheat

• 1/4 cup dried cranberries, or blueberries, raisins, etc.

INSTRUCTIONS

1. Mix all ingredients and let them soak in water for at least 1/2 hour or more.

2. You can also add some fruit juice to the water for added sweetness.

3. Cook 10-15 minutes over a medium-low flame depending on desired thickness.

4. Top with a very light sprinkling of brown sugar, fresh fruit and yogurt.

15. Chocolate Fudge Banana Muffin

INGREDIENTS

• 3large bananas

• ⅔cup granulated sugar

• 1large egg

• ⅓cup unsweetened applesauce

- ½cupwhole-wheat flour, spoon & levelled

- ½cupall-purpose flour, spoon & levelled

- ½cupunsweetened cocoa powder

- ½tspsalt

- 1tspbaking soda

- 1tspbaking powder

- 1cupsemi-sweet chocolate chips, plus more for topping

INSTRUCTIONS

1. Preheat the oven to 375 degrees F. Line a muffin tin with baking cups.

2. Set aside. In a large bowl mash, the bananas with a fork.

Mash them very well – no big lumps. Stir in the sugar, egg, and applesauce.

3. Sift the flour, cocoa powder, salt, baking soda, and baking powder into the wet ingredients. Lightly mix to combine.

4. Fold in chocolate chips. The batter will be a little chunky.

Do not overmix.

5. Divide the batter between the 12 muffin cups – fill them all the way to the top.

6. Bake for 18 to 20 minutes or until a toothpick inserted into the middle comes out clean.

7. Allow muffins to cool for 3 minutes, then transfer to a wire rack to cool completely.

8. Muffins stay fresh in an airtight container at room temperature for up to 5 days.

16. Vegan Teriyaki Tofu Triangles

INGREDIENTS

• 20 oz tofu, firm, pressed

• 2 tbsp soy sauce, reduced-sodium

• 1 tbsp olive oil

• 1 tsp sesame oil

• 1 tbsp honey

• 1 tsp rice vinegar

• ½ tsp ginger, ground

• ½ tsp hoisin sauce

• salt and ground black pepper, to taste

Optional Garnish

• ¼ tsp mixed sesame seeds, toasted

• ¼ tsp green onions, thinly sliced

INSTRUCTIONS

1. Combine sesame oil, honey, rice vinegar, ground ginger, soy sauce, and hoisin sauce.

Mix until evenly incorporated.

2. Season to taste with salt and pepper. Set aside.

3. Cut the tofu into half-thick pieces.

Cut both pieces in half again, so they are ¼ -inch thick, forming the shape of squares.

Slice each piece diagonally to form 2 triangles.

4. Transfer to a shallow pan and coat with sauce.

Marinate for 10 to 15 minutes.

5. In a wide skillet with olive oil over medium-high heat, sear the marinated tofu, turning the side frequently until they are nicely brown.

6. Garnish the tofu with minced onions and sesame seeds.

You can also serve the remaining sauce as well.

17. Sautéed Spinach And Kale

INGREDIENTS

• 3 cups baby spinach, packed

• 2 cups kale, packed

• 2 tbsp olive oil

• 1 tbsp red wine vinegar

• 2 cloves garlic, crushed

• 2 tsp chili flakes

• 1 tsp dried basil

• salt and ground black pepper, to taste

For Garnish:

• chili flakes

INSTRUCTIONS

1. Sauté all of the seasonings and garlic in a skillet for about 4 minutes.

2. Next, add the kale and spinach into the skillet and stir sporadically.

3. Season with salt and pepper. Adjust accordingly.

4. Continue stirring until the greens have wilted and everything is well mixed.

5. Garnish with chili flakes, serve and enjoy!

18. Honey Soy Glazed COD with Quinoa

INGREDIENTS

• 4 cod fillets

• 2 tbsp. honey

• 2 tbsp. soy sauce

• 1 garlic clove, minced

• 1 tbsp. rice wine vinegar

• 1 tsp. sesame seed

- 1 tbsp. lime juice

- 1 ½ cup quinoa

- 3 cups water

- 1 tsp. Salt

- 1 tsp. pepper

INSTRUCTIONS

1. Arrange the cod on a sheet pan and season with black pepper.

2. In a pan, mix the honey, soy sauce, garlic, rice wine vinegar, lime juice, and sesame seeds over medium heat.

3. Bring the pan to a simmer and simmer for 2 minutes before taking the pan off the heat.

4. Bake the cod for 4 minutes.

5. Drizzle some of the honey soy sauce glaze over the cod and bake for 6 more minutes.

6. Drizzle with the rest of the glaze.

7. Meanwhile, mix the quinoa and water in a pot and bring the pot to a boil.

8. Lower the heat, cover the pot, and simmer for 15 minutes.

9. Serve the quinoa with the cod.

19. Peppered Lemon Chicken

INGREDIENTS

• 4 boneless and skinless chicken breasts

• 2 tbsp all-purpose flour

• 1/2 tsp grated lemon zest

• 1/4 tsp fresh ground black pepper

• 1 tbsp extra virgin olive oil

• 2/3 cup reduced sodium chicken broth

• 1 tbsp salted butter

• 1 tbsp fresh parsley

• 2 tsp fresh lemon juice

INSTRUCTIONS

1. Mix the flour, zest, and pepper on a plate.

2. Next, dip each chicken in the flour mixture and coat it on both sides. Make sure to shake off any excess flour.

3. Heat the oil in a large skillet over medium heat, then add the chicken and cook them for 3 to 4 minutes per side.

4. After cooking, remove the chicken from heat.

5. Add the chicken broth to the skillet and bring the contents to a boil.

Stir to scrape up any brown bits.

6. Cook the chicken for 3 minutes.

After that, mix in the butter and remove the chicken from heat.

7. Garnish the chicken with parsley and lemon juice and pour any sauce of your choice over it.

Afterward, serve it hot and enjoy!

20. Grilled Okra

INGREDIENTS

• 1 lb fresh okra

• 1 tbsp dark Asian style sesame oil, or extra virgin olive oil

• salt and pepper

INSTRUCTIONS

1. Preheat the grill to high.

2. Trim the tips off the stems of the okra, but do not cut into the pods.

3. Lay 5 pieces of okra side by side in a neat row at the edge of a cutting board.

4. Skewer crosswise with 2 bamboo skewers, one at the top, one at the bottom.

5. Lightly brush the skewered okra with sesame oil and season with salt and pepper.

6. Grill the okra until tender and lightly browned, 3 to 5 minutes per side, turning once with a flat spatula.

7. Serve the okra at once, letting each guest remove the skewers.

21. Dark Chocolate Avocado Mousse

INGREDIENTS

- 2pcsRipe Avocados

- 4oz70% cacao baking chocolate melted

- ¼cupcocoa powder unsweetened

- ⅓cup almond milk

- ⅓cup maple syrup

- ½tspvanilla extract

- ¼tspground cinnamon

- sea salt

INSTRUCTIONS

1. In a food processor, combine the avocados, melted chocolate, cocoa powder, maple syrup, almond milk, vanilla, cinnamon and a pinch of salt. Puree until creamy.

Spoon the mousse into 4 small ramekins and chill for at least 1 hour.

2. Serve the mousse topped with a dollop of whipped cream and/or your desired toppings.

22. Grilled Salmon

INGREDIENTS

- 2 tbsp extra virgin olive oil

- 2 cloves garlic, chopped

- 1/4 cup basil leaves, chopped

- 2 lemons, juiced

- 1 lb salmon fillet

- 2 tsp salt-free lemon-pepper seasoning

- 2 lb asparagus

INSTRUCTIONS

1. Heat a sauté pan with garlic and olive oil for about 2 minutes until the garlic becomes fragrant.

2. Add basil and, after a while, stop heating the pan.

3. Whisk the basil in lemon juice and set aside.

4. Sprinkle the salmon with lemon-pepper seasoning and set aside.

5. Preheat a covered grill pan with roast asparagus for 3 minutes, shaking occasionally.

6. Brush the salmon with lemon garlic mixture.

7. Place the salmon on the grill pan with the asparagus and cook until the former becomes crusty.

8. Top the cooked asparagus together with the salmon and garlic mixture and serve.

23. Moroccan Lentil Salad

INGREDIENTS

- ½ cup dry lentils

- 1½ cups water

- 7½ oz chickpeas, (½ can) drained

- 2 tomatoes, chopped

- 4 green onions, chopped

- 2 hot green Chile peppers, minced

- 1 green bell pepper, chopped

- ½ yellow bell pepper, chopped

- 1 red bell pepper, chopped

- 1 lime, juiced

- 2 tbsp olive oil

- ¼ cup fresh cilantro, chopped

- salt to taste

INSTRUCTIONS

1. Place lentils and water in a pot. Bring water to boil, reduce to simmer. Cook for 30 minutes or until tender.

2. In a medium size mixing bowl, combine lentils, chickpeas, tomatoes, green onions, green chilies, bell peppers, lime juice, olive oil, cilantro, and salt to taste.

3. Toss well. Chill for 20 minutes. Serve chilled.

24. Deluxe Crockpot Oatmeal

INGREDIENTS

- 2 cups milk

- ¼ cup brown sugar

- 1 tbsp butter, melted

- ¼ tsp salt

- ½ tsp cinnamon

- 1 cup steel-cut oats

- 1 cup apple, finely chopped

- ½ cup raisins, or dates

- ½ cup walnuts, or almonds, chopped

INSTRUCTIONS

1. Grease your crockpot using a non-stick cooking spray and throw in all of your ingredients inside.

2. Give it a quick mix until everything is well incorporated.

3. Cover the crockpot and put it on low heat.

Cook it overnight for 8 to 9 hours.

4. Stir the oatmeal once done.

Top it off with more bananas, raisins, or nuts of your choice and indulge in your delicious crockpot oatmeal!

25. Vinegar-Marinated Green Beans

INGREDIENTS

- 1½ lb green beans

- 1 red onions, small, or sweet onions

- ¼ cup balsamic vinegar

- ½ cup white vinegar

- 1 garlic clove, minced

- ⅛ cup sugar

- 2 tbsp extra-virgin olive oil

- salt, ½ to ¾ tsp

- ½ tsp ground black pepper

INSTRUCTIONS

1. Cook green beans in boiling water for 4 to 5 minutes until tender but still crisp.

2. Drain water and immerse the green beans in ice water till cool.

Drain again afterward.

3. Whisk sugar, white vinegar, olive oil, balsamic vinegar, pepper, and salt, in a serving bowl.

Add onion and green beans and stir together.

4. Marinate in the refrigerator for at least 5 hours or overnight and shake it once in a while before serving!

26. Chickpea Burger

INGREDIENTS

• 2cupsdried chickpeas, (garbanzo beans)

• water, to cover

• ½cupcilantro leaves, and stems, roughly chopped

• 2medium eggs

• 5garlic cloves, peeled

• 3tbspchickpea flour

• 2tbsptahini

• 2tspground coriander

• 1tspsalt

• 1tspground cumin

• ½tspchili powder

• ½cupvegetable oil, or as needed

INSTRUCTIONS

1. Place the chickpeas into a large container, then cover it with several inches of cool water.

2. Let stand for 8 hours to overnight.

3. Drain the water, then transfer the chickpeas to a pot and cover with water.

4. Bring the water to a boil, then reduce the heat and simmer for 1 hour, until chickpeas are tender.

5. Cool chickpeas until easily handled.

6. Combine the chickpeas, cilantro, eggs, garlic, chickpea flour, tahini, coriander, salt, cumin, and chili powder in a blender, then blend until well mixed but still chunky.

7. Form mixture into patties.

8. Heat oil in a large skillet over medium heat.

9. Fry patties for 3 minutes per side, until golden and crisp.

10. Serve, and enjoy!

27. Spaghetti with Mackerel and Pine Nuts

INGREDIENTS

- ¼cupgolden raisins

- 2tbsphot water

- ¾lbspaghetti

- 7tbspolive oil

- 1lbmackerel fillets

- 1tspsalt

- ½tspfresh ground black pepper

- 1small onion

- ¼cuppine nuts

- ¼cupfresh dill, chopped

INSTRUCTIONS

1. Put the raisins and the hot water in a small bowl and leave until the water is absorbed. In a large pot of boiling, salted water, cook the spaghetti for about 12 minutes until just done. Drain the spaghetti.

2. Meanwhile, in a large non-stick frying pan, heat 1 tablespoon of the oil over moderate heat.

Sprinkle the mackerel with ¼ teaspoon each of the salt and pepper.

3. Cook the fish for 2 to 3 minutes per side for ½-inch thick fillets until just done.

Remove the fish and then wipe out the pan. When the fish is cool enough to handle, discard the skin and flake the fish.

4. In the same pan, heat 1 tablespoon of the oil over moderately low heat. Add the onion and cook, stirring, for about 3 minutes until starting to soften.

Add the pine nuts and cook, stirring occasionally, for about 3 minutes until starting to brown.

5. Add the raisins, mackerel, the remaining salt, and pepper. Cook for about 2 minutes until heated through. Toss the mixture with spaghetti, the remaining olive oil, and the dill.

6. Serve and enjoy.

28. Barley Oat Pancakes

INGREDIENTS

- 1cupoat flour

- 1cupbarley flour

- ¼cupwheat germ

- 2tbspbrown sugar

- 1tbspbaking powder

- 1tspsalt

- 1½cupsskim milker as needed

- 2eggsslightly beaten

- ½bananamashed

- 2tbsphoney

- 1tbspoil

- 1tbspvanilla extract

INSTRUCTIONS

1. Mix oat flour, barley flour, wheat germ, brown sugar, baking powder, and salt together in a bowl and make a well in the center.

2. Stir milk, eggs, banana, honey, oil, and vanilla extract together in a separate bowl. Pour milk mixture into the well in the flour mixture and gently stir just until the batter is moistened and slightly lumpy.

3. Heat a griddle or skillet over medium-low heat.

Drop a small amount of water on the surface to test if the griddle is ready.

4. Lightly grease the griddle by running a paper towel dabbed with oil around the bottom of the griddle.

5. Drop batter by large spoonfuls onto the griddle forming 4- inch to 6-inch circles and cook until bubbles form and the edges are dry.

6. Flip and cook until browned on the other side for about 2 to 3 minutes. Repeat with the remaining batter.

29. Simple Roasted Vegetables

INGREDIENTS

- 1smalleggplant

- 1tspsalt

- 4largepotatoes, red-skinned

- 3tbspextra-virgin olive oil

- 1envelopesalad dressing mix

- 2mediumzucchini

- 1mediumred onion

INSTRUCTIONS

1. Position a rack in the top third of the oven and preheat to 425 degrees F.

Lightly oil a large rimmed baking sheet, preferably a 17×13-inch half-sheet pan.

2. Toss the eggplant and salt together in a colander and let stand for 30 minutes to drain off excess bitter juices. Rinse the eggplant well and pat dry with paper towels.

3. Put the potatoes, 1 tablespoon oil, and 1 tablespoon salad dressing mix in a large bowl and toss until the potatoes are coated.

Spread on the baking sheet. Roast for 10 minutes.

4. Put the eggplant, zucchini, and red onion, the remaining oil, and 1 tablespoon of salad dressing mix in the bowl and toss until vegetables are coated.

5. Add the potatoes, mix well, and spread them out.

Roast for about 40 minutes until the vegetables are tender.

6. Serve hot and enjoy.

30. Strawberry and Broccoli Smoothie

INGREDIENTS

- 1 broccoli, serving cut

- 1 cup strawberries, thawed

- 1 cup low-fat milk

- 8 oz apple juice

- 1 banana

• 1 scoop whey protein powder

INSTRUCTIONS

1. Add all ingredients into a blender and blend until smooth.

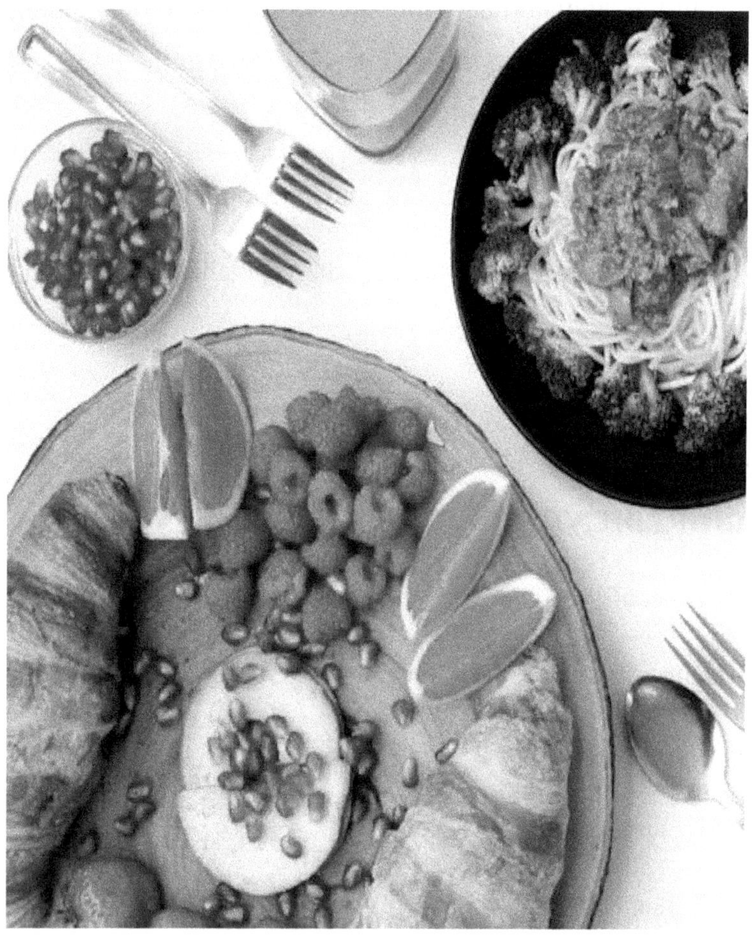

CONCLUSION

This **Blood Cholesterol Diet Cookbook,** embarks not just on a journey of culinary delight but on a path to lifelong health and vitality. Throughout this book, we've explored the profound impact that food choices can have on our cholesterol levels and overall well-being.

By embracing the principles of a cholesterol-conscious diet and harnessing the power of wholesome, nutritious ingredients, you've taken a proactive step towards improving your cardiovascular health.

This cookbook has been crafted to empower you with knowledge and creativity in the kitchen. From hearty breakfasts to satisfying dinners and delightful desserts, each recipe has been meticulously designed to be both delicious and supportive of your health goals.

By incorporating a variety of heart-healthy ingredients such as fiber-rich grains, lean proteins, and antioxidant-packed fruits and vegetables, you've not only learned to manage your cholesterol levels but also to savor every bite.

As you've journeyed through these pages, you've discovered that eating for heart health does not mean sacrificing flavor or enjoyment. Instead, it's about making informed choices that nourish your body and enhance your well-being.

Whether you're preparing a quick weekday meal for yourself or hosting a gathering with loved ones, the recipes in this cookbook offer a wealth of options to suit every occasion and palate.

Beyond the kitchen, **"The Blood Cholesterol Diet Cookbook"** serves as a comprehensive guide to understanding cholesterol and its role in cardiovascular health.

You've learned how to decipher food labels, make mindful grocery choices, and adopt sustainable eating habits that support long-term health benefits. Armed with this knowledge, you are empowered to make informed decisions about your diet and lifestyle, paving the way for a healthier future.

Remember, the journey to better health is not just about what you eat but also about the lifestyle choices you make every day. Incorporating regular physical activity, managing stress levels, and maintaining a positive outlook are all integral components of a holistic approach to cardiovascular wellness.

By embracing these principles alongside the delicious recipes found in this cookbook, you are taking proactive steps towards achieving optimal health and vitality.

As you continue on your journey, **let "The Blood Cholesterol Diet Cookbook"** remain a trusted companion in your quest for better health.

Whether you're embarking on a new chapter in your wellness journey or simply seeking inspiration in the kitchen, may these recipes continue to nourish your body, uplift your spirit, and bring joy to your table.

Here's to a future filled with vibrant health, delicious meals, and the satisfaction of knowing you're taking control of your well-being—one delicious bite at a time.

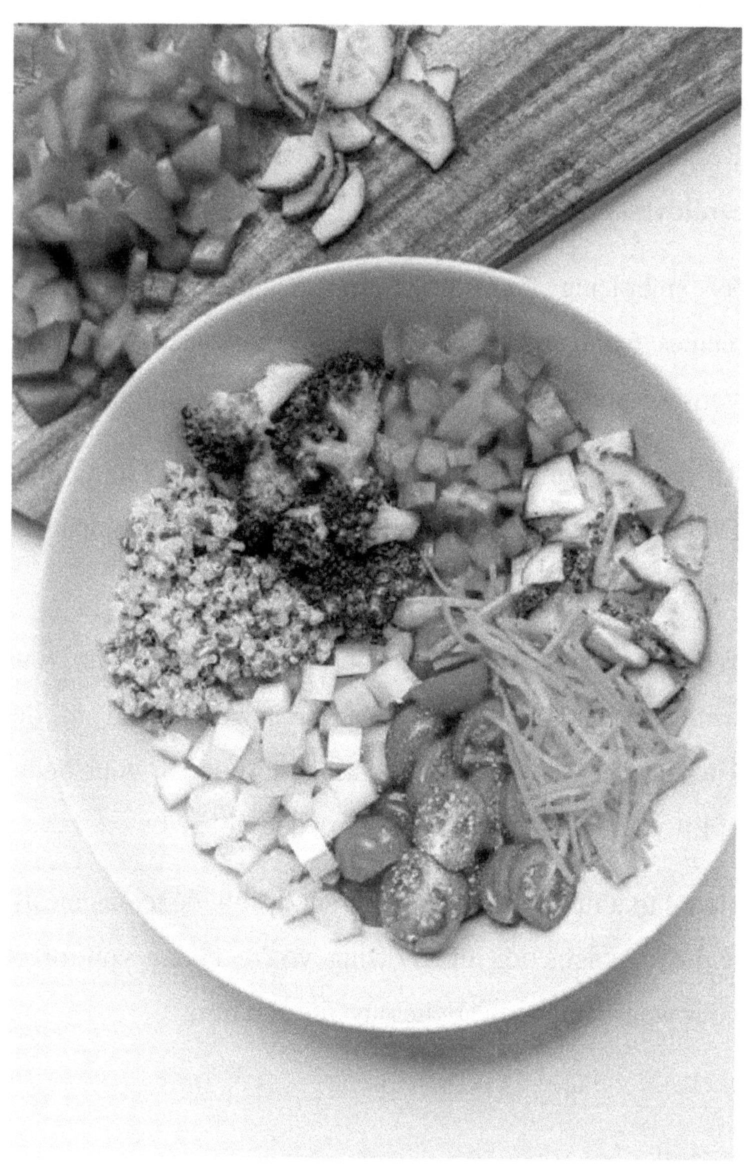